CW00434255

PRESENTED TO

_____

BY

_____

ON

_____

U.G.L.Y.

U Gotta Love Yourself

It's Your Time to Fly

What if you are supposed to be great?

Would you linger and still procrastinate?

What if you were supposed to shine?

Would you say I will now take what's mine?

What if you are supposed to be a star?

Would you go farther no matter how far?

What if you stopped asking yourself why?

Then today you decide it's your time to fly.

Ten Ways to Love Yourself

You must be a priority. **11**

You must study for you. **19**

You must have me time. **28**

You must include God. **36**

You must get rid of bad habits. **43**

You must have play time. **51**

You must take care of your business. **59**

You must take care of you. **64**

You must forgive yourself. **69**

You must be around good people. **73**

Introduction

Stop! Before you decide this book is not for you ask yourself these three questions:

1) Am I always taking care of everybody else?

2) Do I feel guilty when I am trying to relax because I feel I always have more work to do?

3) Do I always take "working vacations"?

If you answered yes to any of these questions, then this book is for you. Also, if you have been called a workaholic, told you need to slow down, or are overwhelmed by stress then this book is for you.

How can this book help?

You can be the hero. However, this book lets you examine how you do it. This book is not about telling "Superman" to stop being "Super" or "Wonder Woman" to stop being the "Wonder" that she is. It's about letting you know how to fight the "villains", take care of your family, and show your love for God.

3 Day Journey

This book is designed to be read in three days. Consider reading this book as your weekend retreat, which can occur on Friday, Saturday, Sunday or any three days of the week. Reading this book takes only a short amount of time but the wisdom of this book is timeless. Each day (chapter) of this book is set up in this manner:

1) Advice

2) Prayer

3) Summary

4) Discussion Questions

Why I Wrote This Book

Her beautiful brown eyes had a tear glaze as she focused them on me. As our eyes met her gaze pieced my soul and shattered my heart into many pieces.

Another set of eyes fixed on me with puzzlement and shouted at me "what is going on!"

Then I was suffocated and shackled with the fear that consumed the whole room.

No one said a word. Then a third set of eyes stared at me. I was not sure what that look was from that last pair of eyes. Maybe anger or fear. No, I think it was disappointment.

Maybe I should say something, but I didn't know what to say. I needed to say something, but my body felt so strange. My heart ached. My head pounded. My arm felt as if I had banged it with a sledge hammer.

And the bed was cold. "Focus, Abe, focus"! I needed to focus on the issue at hand. How do I comfort the woman I love and my babies, my two daughters after doctors have said that I appeared to have had a heart attack?

I needed to say something. I am supposed to be their protector, provider, and the one that made promises come true. Am I a fraud? Am I not the robot that can work and does not need any rest, relaxation, or release?

Is it over? It can't be over. I'm only forty. No! It's not over so man up and say something to let them know you are still the one they can count on, the one who makes things happen.

"Girls, daddy is going to be all right." "The doctor's need to do a test to check out my heart."

"Stac, I got to get back to work." "I can't be laying here on vacation. I'm behind on my work."

"Stac can you let my job know I don't think I will be back to finish up today, but I will come in tomorrow and get caught up?"

If looks could kill my lovely wife would be on death row because she just murdered me.

Then my wife told me in many, many, many words over an extended period that I had a problem loving me. I honestly never thought about that because I needed to always take care of somebody else. So, I have to look at the scriptures to figure this out. These principles are mentioned by Jesus in Matthew 22:37-40 and will be the focus of this book, UGLY.

"And He said to him, 'You shall love the Lord your God with all your heart, and with all your soul, and with all your mind.' This is the great and foremost commandment. The second is like it, You shall love the Lord your neighbor as yourself.'"

Day 1

Yourself by Loving God

Dear Me, Myself, and I,

I love myself. Yes, I do. But there are so many people who are "blue". Counseling and coaching day after day. It's hard to not work and get away. Life is filled with so many things to do. How can I have time for me, myself, and I too? I pray to God for all the world each day. I love God almighty in every way. I go to church. I serve and help those in need. I also teach to plant the seed. My body is weary, and I seek some peace. But I know that won't come until I'm deceased.

Sincerely,

Us

You must be a priority.

"Do you love yourself?"

A single tear streamed down her face as she slowly shook her head from side to side. "No." she relied softly.

As I heard the single word she spoke, her feeling of despair enveloped the room. I could feel her pain screaming out at me. As a counselor in the detox department, I had heard this answer many times, but the initial force of the sting pricks my heart every time.

I wish I could say that this was confined to a few who were experiencing the pains of withdrawal from substances. However, I find some of my friends and family suffer quietly without the feeling that they are worthy of self-love.

Then, I turn the mirror on myself. Do I love me? Since love is an action word, do I truly express self-love? Or am I a hypocrite that peddles shallow words to patients but do not show it through my actions? Do I love me is the million-dollar question? Right now, I would have to say maybe but my actions would probably answer no.

It took losing almost everything that I had worked so hard for to realize this. I never thought I should be a priority because I felt I was put on this earth to help others. I did not really need much to survive. If I had just enough to make it, then I was all right. However, there was a monkey wrench in this plan. I got married and had a family. Even if I felt that just enough was ok, my wife did not feel that way. Growing up poor like I did allows you to get use to not having much. I was comfortable with not being comfortable.

I never really had anything, so it did not bother me to not have a lot. At first, I decided that my compromise would be to work a lot of hours to make extra money. I know how to work, and nobody could out work me. So, I spent most of my adult life working 80, 90, 100 + hours a week. I would send money to my mom at first. After getting married, I realized that I did not make enough money to support our family's lifestyle. So, I worked a lot. Then we had two daughters. And, I still worked a lot.

Work, Church, Family, Work. Work, Church, Work, Family, Work. Work, Work, Family, Work, Church, Work. Although I worked more and more, we never had enough except when I ran a strict budget and paid most things myself. Again, I am used to not having much. The amount of money that I was making was more than I ever had. Day after day I worked and worked. Every day was the same and we never had enough money. Then I began to reflect and think about what I was doing. Do I really believe that I am a priority? I admit that sometimes I forget that I am a priority to God. The Bible reminds me of that in Matthew 6:25-32:

[25] "Therefore I say to you, do not worry about your life, what you will eat or what you will drink; nor about your body, what you will put on. Is not life more than food and the body more than clothing? [26] Look at the birds of the air, for they neither sow nor reap nor gather into barns; yet your heavenly Father feeds them. Are you not of more

value than they? ²⁷ Which of you by worrying can add one cubit to his stature?

²⁸ "So why do you worry about clothing? Consider the lilies of the field, how they grow: they neither toil nor spin; ²⁹ and yet I say to you that even Solomon in all his glory was not arrayed like one of these. ³⁰ Now if God so clothes the grass of the field, which today is, and tomorrow is thrown into the oven, will He not much more clothe you, O you of little faith?³¹ "Therefore do not worry, saying, 'What shall we eat?' or 'What shall we drink?' or 'What shall we wear?' ³² For after all these things the Gentiles seek. For your heavenly Father knows that you need all these things.

God loves us and care for us. There was a time when I was a child that I felt that nobody loved me. I gained a lot of comfort when I realized that God loved me and would take care of me. Since you know that God loves you and makes you a priority, it only makes sense for you to make Him a priority in your life. You must value you before anyone else will.

What is most important in your life? If God is most important, then put Him first. Jesus says in *Matthew 6:33, "But seek first His kingdom and His righteousness, and all these things will be added to you."* This verse helps to determine what our priority should be. God should be first. God should be first in everything we do. God should be first in every aspect of our lives. A good place to start putting God first is in your schedule.

Yes, you have a multitude of commitments, duties, and

obligations. Yet, you should not leave God out in the abundance of the things that have to be done. God is needed now more than ever. But you must make sure your schedule gives adequate time to cultivate your relationship with God. God must be a priority. If He is, then He should be a major part of your schedule and not get just the leftovers.

Sometimes, the only way to make God a part of your schedule is to make sure you schedule time to spend seeking God. Make sure the time you spend with God is quality and not just quantity.

Put God first and He will bless you. This is the bonus. Make no mistake that you should put God first because you love Him. In "The Purpose Driven Life", Rick Warren starts the book by saying that it is not us, it is about Him. We must remember that our goal is to follow God.

But wait! How can God be first if we are a priority? Putting God first does not mean that we neglect ourselves. Contrary to what many may think, the better we take care of ourselves spiritually, mentally, and physically, the better we can serve God.

Think about it. The better spiritually we are the more we can be a light for Jesus. The better mentally we are, the better we can think of ways to praise Him. The better physically we are, the better we can lift our hands to show that we glorify Him.

You are taught to make goals to achieve academic and career success but then some of us fail to make real spiritual goals. Take time to make spiritual goals. Do you have a goal to become a Bible class teacher? What about learning a Bible verse? How will your career goals affect your spiritual goals?

Remember that God is ready and willing to bless you. All you must do is put Him first. Often, we miss our blessing because we focus so much on what is not going right. We focus on the trials, the troubles, and the tribulations. Just remember that you serve a Savior that can walk on water, a Savior that is able to turn water to wine, and a Savior that is able to calm any storm. So, do not focus on the storm. Focus on Jesus and serve Him.

Make service a priority. I remember when I was about to graduate from college, the transmission went out on my car. I was quoted prices well over a thousand dollars to get a new transmission. At the time, I was a struggling college student and had very, little money. I remember some of the men of the congregation that I was attending decided to get together and fix my car.

Not only that, but since my car broke down in a place over four hours away, they rented a dolly and one of the men got up early one morning and picked up my car. They said that this was my graduation present from them. When I was told about this plan, I really did not want them to do this because I thought it was too much.

Then one of the men said something that I will always remember. He said, "Don't mess up my blessing." He went on to elaborate that because he was doing something good for me, God would bless him. Now I know this is true. It is when we stretch out our hands to help someone that our same hands are opened to receive blessings from God.

It is when we help others, we make a connection with Jesus. Matthew 25:35-40 says, "For I was hungry, and you gave Me something to eat; I was thirsty, and you gave Me something to drink; I was a stranger, and you invited Me in; naked, and you clothed Me; I was sick, and you visited Me; I was in prison and you came to Me. Then the righteous will answer Him, 'Lord when did we see You hungry, and feed You, or thirsty and give You something to drink?' And when did we see You a stranger, and invite You in, or naked and clothe You? When did we see You sick, or in prison, and come to You?' The King will answer and say to them, 'Truly I say to you, to extent that you did it to one of these brothers of Mine, even the least of them, you did it to Me.'

Yes, when we serve others, we are serving Jesus. We must remember that Jesus lived a life of service. No matter whether you are at work, school, or meeting for worship you should have a desire to serve. I mention worship because we sometimes forget that when we meet for worship, we have great opportunities to provide service to others.

It is important to note that worship and service are used together so many times in the Bible. We need to attend worship services. When you worship God, you show your love and adoration. God loves us so much. Shouldn't we show Him how much we love Him through our praise to Him?

I know some of you say I can worship God anywhere.

What is the big deal about going to a church building? Well, we must remember that we are a family. When we come together, we can encourage one another (Hebrews 10:24, 25). You may say with so many obligations, it is so easy not to attend because you do not have time.

However, you must make attending services a priority. A loving congregation can be a lot of encouragement for a troubled soul. I am so surprised that people feel that they do not need to assemble with other Christians. In Psychology class, we learn that we have a need to belong.

I believe this is true and may be the reason that God instructs us to meet. I can only imagine what consolation it must have been for Christians who were being persecuted to meet. It must have been great comfort in knowing that someone else understood the trials, tribulations, and troubles. God has instituted a support group called the church. So, take advantage of it.

If you understand serving others, then you have to be willing to also be served by others. You must remember that you are important to God. Therefore don't forget to make yourself a priority and make sure you fill your cup also. Don't forget to love you! Don't forget to take care of you! Don't forget in order to love your neighbor as yourself that you have to love yourself!

There is an event that happened when I was a teenager that sticks with me. I heard a crash in the bathroom that was immediately followed by a moaning sound like a wounded big dog that refused to lay down after receiving a fatal blow. I rushed to the bathroom and opened the cracked door to see my grandfather on his knees over the toilet.

"Are you ok?" I asked clearly knowing he was not ok.

This proud man shook his head yes, he was ok, but it was appearance to my high school eyes that he was suffering so I went to get my mom.

My grandfather kept yelling he was all right, but he could not get up. He had worked all day in the fields. He could out work anybody. And now, "Superman" could not get up.

This was the first time in my life that I realized my grandfather was not invincible. It was the first time I realized that even he had some type of kryptonite. It was the first time that I realized that my grandfather was mortal. Amazingly, my mom, my superhero, my "Storm" used to always warn me about working too much.

She would say...

"Abraham, don't do like I did when I was young."

"I overworked myself the death and had a nervous breakdown."

"Don't you work yourself into a nervous breakdown!"

"That money ain't worth it!"

Self-care matters. Self-care is not selfish. Self-care is a necessity. So please make it a priority or learn it the hard way.

You must study for you.

"Down goes Lewis." Like a prize fighter receiving the knockout punch I went down.

I laid on the floor dazed. My vision was blurry. I struggled to breathe.

Where is my inhaler? Where is my inhaler, I thought?

As I fumbled and bumbled through my pockets for that inhaler, I could feel myself fading as the energy escaped my body.

Finally, my fingers located that vital appendage that most asthmatics have grown accustom to living with because of times like these. My fingers, my fingers are not working right.

I knew then that I only had a few seconds before my body turned itself off and the light in my brain would go to darkness.

"God help me!" "God help me, make my fingers move."

With every ounce of my being, I prayed and focused on moving two fingers. At last, my fingers moved. Two of my fingers locked unto the inhaler with an unbelievable vise grip.

Somehow like magic the inhaler popped out of my pocket. Half the battle was won now.

God, I need you!

Somehow my hand was able to find my mouth. Thank God for my big lips. As my lips maneuvered the top off the inhaler, I pressed the button and did my best to inhale but I had nothing left. I pressed again as the inhaler fell out of my mouth. It was over.

As my body tensed and I laid there, I waited to go into nothingness. I gasped for air like a fish out of water. Now no more fighting. It was time to give into the extreme exhaustion.

As I relaxed, I heard a knock at the door. The knock jolted me out of my trance. Then someone came in. It was Stacey. Without hesitation, she asked what was wrong. I said, "Let me catch my breath".

She immediately called EMS. Unfortunately, I had said the exact phrase that my patient in the Emergency Room said to me before he took his last breaths and died and could not be resuscitated.

EMS came and I was taken to the hospital. They said that I had but a few hours left. At the time, I was a nurse technician and I had worked about ninety hours in six days. I was used to that, but I had eaten very little because I had no money. I had sent my money home to help my mom buy food.

So, I was dehydrated, exhausted, and asthmatic. My body was like a car that had run out of gas.

I learned the hard way about overworking myself and not eating right. I have a brother who has been encouraging me to improve on these issues. I learned some things from that incident, and it caused me to make some changes in my life. I must take time to fill my cup up physically, mentally, and spiritually or suffer some severe consequences.

Even in college, I took steps to fill my cup up physically, mentally, and spiritually. Things were not going well for me at the University of South Carolina. My body was battered, my mind felt tattered, and I just needed a fresh start to regroup. So, I switch to a smaller school and decided to change my major. I packed up and moved to Fayetteville, North Carolina.

What a difference this change made! Things were going so well at Methodist College. Then I received a phone call. My grandfather had passed, and I needed to go to the funeral. I also knew this would be a struggle for my mom who was a "daddy's girl".

My grandfather dying sent my mom into a period of permanent melancholy. I would talk to her on the phone and make periodic visits but then my car broke down. I had to rely mainly on phone calls, but I could tell that something just was not right. I convinced my mom to go get help. She did. She stayed a few days in inpatient treatment. For a few weeks, she was a little better. Then she began to get sad again. I would try to comfort her as often as I could in between my studies.

Then again, I asked her to get help. She did. She again received inpatient treatment. She again came out a little better but then things started to progress again in a negative direction. As this happened, she became more and more abusive on the phone. She would get like that when I was home and then it would eventually pass. I was always told that my mom had nerve problems. I never knew what the diagnosis was I just knew that sometimes she would get terribly upset, sometimes confused, and I had learned how to navigate this landmine of emotions from years of experience.

Nerve problems had caused me many sleepless nights. Nerve problems had caused me to be yelled at more times than I could remember. Nerve problems had caused me to be accused of something I did not do and just take it. I was good at taking verbal abuse. She would eventually come back around to being ok and I would be able to reason with her.

But this time she did not get better. This time I had no power to reason with her. This time was different and was spiraling out of control. Fortunately, there was a winter break. Fortunately, my Aunt Mary was there to help me. Fortunately, mental health worked with me.

This was the first time I had to start the process for an involuntary commitment. This was the first time that I started to figure out what was going on. This was the first time I was given the name of the disorder she was being treated for, Schizophrenia.

My mom received treatment. My mom also would now receive her medication by injection once a month. When my mom came out of inpatient treatment, she was so much better. I would talk to her most days on the phone. Every so often or if I thought there was a problem, I would have to come to check on her. I was about two hours away with no working car but fortunately one of my college professors, Dr. John Sill would bring me home to check on my mom.

During the time I was struggling to deal with all that was going on with my mom. I met a family that was sent by God. The Jenkins family was there for me. Sister Linda Jenkins my "Superwoman" always had words of encouragement. She had a superpower that made life seem better after I spoke to her. She constantly reminded me to study my Bible and I saw her studying and applying Biblical principles. She became my mother figure during the time I was in Fayetteville. Momma Jenkins always let me know how important it was to study God's word. Now you do not have to read from paper and print because there is a Bible App.

I used to carry around a pocket Bible. However, on my phone a Bible application has made that unnecessary. We can miss many blessings when we fail to open the "pages" of the Bible. Many of us underestimate the power of the word of God. The Bible has power to change a person. The Bible gives you a guide to go by in life. The Bible offers us a roadmap to heaven. If we want to get to heaven, we must simply follow the instructions that are printed on its pages. If heaven is important to us, then we need to study the roadmap---the Bible.

Do not just say I am going to read my Bible for one hour today. Have a purpose. Let the words of the Bible speak to you. Read with the purpose of trying to improve your life. Study to get close to God.

You must make time to study the Bible. Put it in your

schedule. Set your priorities. If God is your top priority, then it makes sense to want to know more about God. You can learn more about God by reading the Bible. The Bible tells you how you should live while on earth. It is your compass that points to heaven.

My suggestion to you is to find a time that works best for your schedule to study the Bible. For some, studying the Bible first thing in the morning works. For others, it may be in the evening. Decide how much time you want to spend and just do it.

Be systematic about how you study God's word. Today there are several good devotional Bibles that break the Bible up into small sections often with author's comments and his interpretation of what he gets from the passage.

Do not just take it at face value. Make sure you study, question, meditate, and pray about what the passage means. Search the scriptures yourself.

Also, there are Bible reading plans that give you a plan to read the entire Bible in a year or the New Testament in a year. Surprisingly, to read the entire Bible in a year, you will only have to read a few chapters a day.

There are some good Bible Apps or Internet sites that will give you yearly Bible reading plans. Some will even allow you to create a plan from the current day to customize your plan for a year. To read the New Testament in a year, you may be able to do so by spending only ten to fifteen minutes a day reading.

Finally, one of my favorite methods is the topical study. This is where you choose a topic and search the Bible to see what it has to say about a specific topic. For instance, you may use a Bible concordance or an internet site to find out how many times the Bible uses a certain word. A word study may enhance your understanding of a word.

I especially find it helpful to study an issue or word that I am currently dealing with. The issue may be worry or anger. The Bible has the answers to every issue that you are dealing with in life. After I find what the Bible has to say, I can apply what I read to my life.

The Bible is better than any self-help book that you can find because it presents God's help for problems. I believe that we accomplish much more when we are God helped. Studying the Bible will allow you to understand how to receive God's help.

But you must make time to read the Bible. Here is a suggestion. Steal a little time by putting a Bible App on your phone. During moments you may be waiting in line read a few verses. You will be pleased to find how much you can read during these moments. Instead of being upset about having to wait, be productive. Doing this may not only change your day, it could change your life.

Top Ten Reasons Biblical Moses Could Be a Social Media Influencer Today

10) He wrote on tablets.

9) He had many followers.

8) He loved his followers.

7) He made special appearances to his followers.

6) He spent a lot of time chatting with his followers.

5) He had a rock hit.

4) He wrote 5 books.

3) He starred in a movie (The Ten Commandment).

2) He had sponsorship (God).

1) His followers had a watch party for him.

You do not have to be Moses to be an influencer. Following God's word can make you someone that others come to for advice.

The Bible offers help for making decisions in life. You can learn from the commandments that are stated. There are also many examples of people making both good and bad decisions.

Reading the Bible can help you be successful in life. The book, The Richest Man Who Ever Live, demonstrates how Steven Scott used principles from the book of Proverbs to propel him to become a millionaire. I am not saying that reading the Bible will make you a millionaire. I am saying that you will achieve great riches far more than money if you follow the Bible's principles. Therefore, if you want success in life, you need to open God's Word.

You must have me time.

Mrs. Linda English is my "Wonder Woman" and was at one time my work mom. She is my mentor. She has been my mediator. She has been willing to give her time to help me be better. I have learned so much from her. She taught me the concept of me time. Often during her lunch, she would go to her car or find some quiet spot to be alone. It did not have to be long, maybe thirty minutes. She liked that time. She considered it an essential part of her day.

This time usually came during the middle part of her day. She would come back recharged, refreshed, and ready to complete the rest of the day. This was part of her everyday work routine. Her actions taught me so much about self-care.

She taught me no matter how hard you work for everybody else that you need to make some time to work on yourself. She taught me that there is value in being self-aware. She taught me it is so important to know your strengths as well as your weaknesses.

If I write down all the things, I learned from my Momma English, I would be writing for the rest of my life. I am a better person because of her. I met Momma English during a time when I was working around 90 hours a week and I was not sleeping much. She constantly warned me that this was not a good idea. She told me that I needed to do something different and would give wise suggestions. I love her for being willing to take me under her wings and doing her best to teach me to fly.

"Be still" (Psalm 46:10). A simple phrase but it seems increasingly hard to do. We have truly become a busy, overscheduled, fast paced society. It can be so hard to slow down, to be still. But you need to be able to do this.

A time of solitude gives you an opportunity to be still. This is a time in which you withdraw yourself from the rest of the world to spend time alone with God.

Solitude improves attitude because it allows you to put things in the right prospective. When you spend time in solitude, remember this phrase: Your will be done. This is a phrase that Jesus used when He was dealing with the anguish of the impending cruelty of the cross. This is the best example how we should live and face trials and tribulations.

You may experience some hard times. You may be struggling. You may have some classes that are so challenging that you sometimes think there is no way you can get your degree. But there is hope.

In the mist of your struggles, storms, and situations God is there for you. You have a "secret weapon" so powerful this world cannot harness it or even fully understand its capabilities. You have a force that can move mountains. You have a direct line of communication to God known as prayer.

Prayer is your opportunity to converse with God. He is listening. Use times of solitude to pause and hear what message God seeks to reveal to you. When you are with God, make sure that you are listening. You can be confident that God is listening to you.

Remember that God is able to win the battle when all seems lost. God is able to be your armor of protection when the enemy wages war against you. God is able to move mountains that you are trying to climb. God unleashes this power when we pray to Him. Therefore, we should never neglect to pray.

So, do not underestimate the power of spending time with God. David proclaimed that he meditated on the words of the Lord both day and night (Psalms 1:2). In solitude, you can do this, and you can be blessed by doing so. I also believe that we should want to spend time with God because of all he has done for us.

Me time allows you to remember that you belong to God. You are his special creation. God loves you. If you do not believe, just look in His book.

John 3:16 New King James Version (NKJV)
16 For God so loved the world that He gave His only begotten Son, that whoever believes in Him should not perish but have everlasting life.

Romans 5:7-8 New King James Version (NKJV)
7 For scarcely for a righteous man will one die; yet perhaps for a good man someone would even dare to die. 8 But God demonstrates His own love toward us, in that while we were still sinners, Christ died for us.

2 Corinthians 12:9-10 New King James Version (NKJV)

[9] And He said to me, "My grace is sufficient for you, for My strength is made perfect in weakness." Therefore most gladly I will rather boast in my infirmities, that the power of Christ may rest upon me. [10] Therefore I take pleasure in infirmities, in reproaches, in needs, in persecutions, in distresses, for Christ's sake. For when I am weak, then I am strong.

Psalm 139:14 New King James Version (NKJV)

[14] I will praise You, for [a] I am fearfully and wonderfully made; Marvelous are Your works, And that my soul knows very well.

Isaiah 64:8 New King James Version (NKJV)

[8] But now, O Lord, You are our Father; We are the clay, and You our potter; And all we are the work of Your hand.

Ephesians 2:10 New King James Version (NKJV)

[10] For we are His workmanship, created in Christ Jesus for good works, which God prepared beforehand that we should walk in them.

Knowing these things allow me to be kind to myself. What is my self-talk like? Would I be comfortable saying what I say to myself to my best friend? Am I saying positive words to me or am I tearing me down? I have to remember that me time has to be constructive and not destructive.

Don't spend your me time in negative dialog. This is a time to listen to your feelings and try to understand you. Me time is about self-awareness. Me time is a time to be honest. It's a time to be authentic. It's a time to be real. In order to love ourselves we have to really know who we are.

--Our Father,

Thank You for choosing to love us despite us. May Your love continue to comfort us. Teach us to be thankful for all you have given us. Help us to love You with all our heart. We also ask You to show us how to love ourselves. For You are the One who loves us best. We pray in the name of Jesus. Amen

Summary

- You must be a priority.

- You must study for you.

- You must have me time.

Discussion Questions

1) What activities are you spending most of your time doing?

2) Do you make time for God in your schedule?

3) Do you have me time?

4) How often do you study the Bible for you?

5) Do you take time to pray each day?

Day 2

Love Yourself by Loving Others

I Love You

A man spends time planning his life

Taking chances and making a sacrifice

But all through the struggles in life I endure

I find myself loving you even more

When I search for words to express how I feel

In time my actions must show I am for real

Loving a woman as beautiful as you

Makes a common man want to say I do

You make love an easy task

I pray to God that our love will last

Looking forward and pressing through time

I picture you and I together a love so divine

Forever to you I will be true

Stacey, I love you

You must include God.

You complete me. It was a great phrase in the movie, Jerry McGuire. I have seen the idea of a significant other completing someone turn into an unrealistic reality in some relationships. For instance, sometimes we fail to do the work to make ourselves better because we want to rely on someone else to do the work for us.

My wife, Stacey, is my self-proclaimed "Invisible Girl". She is the one behind the scenes of everything I do. She is the one that puts a force field of protection around our family. She teaches me every day that God must be included. Although she can get on my last nerve and sometimes, really a lot of times I do not understand her, I always know she is standing on God's side. There is never a question about whether she is going to follow God. We think differently. We approach things differently. However, we agree that God must be included in all we do. God must be included in every relationship.

Remember the Golden Rule. *"Treat others the way you want to be treated"* (Luke 6:31). I remember the acts of kindness that were shown to me by people who loved me. I remember briefly telling a lady about my plight at a church function. I only mentioned some of the highlights almost in passing. A few days later, I remember getting a check in the mail from her and other checks followed for several months. These checks helped me get back on my feet and I will always be grateful.

Over the years, I had tried to be the best giver I could be. However, I learned that sometimes in life that it becomes your time to be a receiver. God has a way of working things out so that both the giver and receiver are blessed.

Also include God in dating relationships. Let me share what dating could lead to. It was Valentine's Day 2001; this day changed my life. I waited outside with one million thoughts running through my head. How would she answer? How would she respond? I had gotten up early and took the hour and half drive to her parents' house.

I had put a dozen lavender roses (purple her favorite color) in front of the door. I had placed three red helium-filled balloons on the sidewalk that was held down with chocolate. There was just one word printed on each of the three balloons. The words were "Will You Marry". And in my hand, I held a fourth balloon that had the word "Me" on it. I held the balloon in one hand, and I had the ring in the other hand.

Now I stood there waiting outside for her to come to the door and come outside. When she opened the door, the first thing she saw was the flowers. She walked down the sidewalk as the balloons led her to me. I dropped to one knee. I had some words from my heart to say but I struggled to get them out. I do remember asking her will you marry me. Time stood still for a moment as I waited for her response as she stood there in her footy pajamas. She said yes.

Asking Stacey to marry me has been one of the best decisions that I have made in my life. Stacey and I started dating when we were in college. She had been my best friend for several years. We grew up together. We went to the same congregation since we were in middle school. Amazingly, our relationship progressed into a beautiful marriage.

Relationships matter. We need others; therefore, we can also conclude that others need us. We must maintain a proper balance of give and take for the relationship to work. Sometimes in life, we will need to be takers, but it should not be all the time. We all have something to offer. We must consider this in all the relationships that we have including the ones of a romantic nature.

Dating presents challenges for Christians. There are certain things that you should consider before you go on a date with anyone. First, you should ask yourself if the person you are considering dating is someone who loves God. Is this person a Christian?

We sometimes take our broken selves and link up with someone that has the same or worst broken issues. There is nothing wrong with finding someone that helps you. However, just do not look for someone to do the work you should complete yourself.

The activities that Christians do on a date and the activities that people who are not Christians do on a date can be vastly different. You want to make sure you are with someone who will help you uphold the morals that you have as a Christian. There can be positive peer pressure on you to do the right thing when the other person is also trying to do the right thing.

The person you date may be the person you marry. It is

hard enough for the marriage to survive with two Christians. So, do not give yourself the potential of going into one where you are the only Christian. You say that people change. The truth is that only the word of God can change anyone.

However, God gives people the chance to make up his or her mind on if they are going to change or not. People tend to change on their time, and some do not want to change. They will be the same for the rest of their lives. So, keep this in mind when you decide to date someone.

There are so many temptations to consider. On a typical date a college student may become drunk, attend a wild party, and have sex on the same night. It is important to be with someone who not only may respect you because you do not do these things but someone who lives the life you live and is abstaining from these things. Who you are with can influence you to sin or not to sin? Choose your relationships wisely.

Even though the woman of my dreams had always been in front of me, timing and circumstances dictated that we did not get into a romantic relationship until the last few years of college. We wandered through the wilderness a while before eventually finding the promise land.

In college, I was called smart and I became amazingly comfortable approaching anyone. I became more of a people person because I was among other people that had goals and found people who shared similar passions. I found a group of friends who will be a part of my journey in life until I die.

For others college proves to be a reality check. I know people who were the best thing since sliced bread at their high school but struggle to adjust in college because they are just another boy or girl. In college nobody considered them to be anything special. A college Christian must be able to adjust to a new environment.

How do you develop the right relationships? First and foremost, make your closest friends, people who love God. This should also be extended to anyone that you are dating.

If you are a Christian, it helps you to be around other Christians. Yes, we do have a responsibility to reach out to those who are not Christians, but I suggest to you that the people you call confidants, the people that you call your advisors, and the people that you want to be around you must be Christians.

I had plenty of people who were not Christians around me, and I consider some of them to be friends. Often, they would come to me for advice. But when I needed guidance, most of the time, I went to my Christian friends because a large portion of my life needed advice that also considered the spiritual. It is hard for someone who is not a Christian to adequately consider the spiritual aspects of a decision.

The Bible is also truly clear when it says that bad company corrupts good morals (1 Corinthians 15:33). There were certain things that my Christians friends were not going to do that my friends who were not Christians had no problem doing. When you are in college, you are away from the watchful eye of your parents.

Therefore, you need people who share the same Christian values. These people can help you make good choices. Even then you will still make some bad decisions. The thing that I knew about my Christian friends was that they were trying to do the right thing just as I was even when we made a bad choice. Often, the bad decisions that we made were due to being young and inexperienced.

The way to develop these relationships is that you be real. Do all you can to be a real Christian every day, 24/7? People are often compelled to help those who are trying to do the right thing. Also, be grateful for everything people do for you. Do not act like people owe you anything or expect people to do things for you. Do all you can and accept help when you need it.

Most importantly, become a giver. Do not always have your hand opened to receive but lend that hand to someone who needs help. The best way to cultivate long lasting relationships is to be someone that people can count on.

My mom is the best giver I know. My mom will give her last to someone if she thinks they need help. Unfortunately, people have sometimes taken advantage of her kindness. Sometimes I would give my mom money to help her, but sometimes she would give that money to someone else because they told her they needed help.

Then she would have to ask someone else for the money she needed. I was on constant watch of this. Sometimes I would have to go pay the bill myself instead of giving the money to my mom. Things were ok but never great for years with me trying to manage things by phone and limited visits. For a long time, the situation stayed about the same. Then things changed with my mom's health and mental state. As life would have it, I was also going through my own personal crisis.

You must get rid of bad habits.

I started to feel sick all the time. My chest, my legs, my left arm, my head, and my back all started to betray me. My leg would gush blood in between jobs. Some mornings the blood would shoot from my leg and splatter on the bathroom wall. It would take all my previous EMT training to stop the bleeding. Then I also injured my back. I have always had some back issues but now my back hurts daily.

I was also struggling at work. My doctor was telling me to slow down. How can I slow down when things are not going well at work? I needed more money for bills. I was losing my mojo and felt as if life was oozing out of my body slowly. I needed to get rid of some bad habits.

In Hebrew 12:1 it tells us to lay aside the weight of sin. We need to let sin go. We need to release sin. If we can do this, we will receive a victory greater than anything this world can offer. As a college student, you have forces approaching you from every direction.

You must be careful. You must be aware of how easy it is to get swept up in something that you never thought you would do. You must keep your eyes open. Don't underestimate the power of Satan. Satan has been scheming people since the beginning of time. He is very experienced at tricking men and women. He is an expert at his craft. Don't think for a second that you are so strong that you will never allow Satan to use you.

The good news is that we serve Jesus who has defeated Satan and left us with instructions on how to win. The

Bible is not only our roadmap, but it is our playbook to win in the game Satan tries to play.

My other mom, Yvonne (a.k.a. my mother-in-law), is my "She-Ra". She has always been willing to lend a helping hand. She has always been willing to lend of her time. And she has always been willing to lend advice whether you want it or not. I have received a lot of good things to take hold of from her. She constantly taught me about the value of being obedient and faithful to God. She taught me that we must do the right thing. She taught me that living God's way is the best way to live.

However, if we are not careful, we can fall into temptations. Fortunately, the Bible helps us understand how to deal with sin through examples and instruction. Consider these examples.

Samaritan Woman at the Well

John 4:4-26 New King James Version

⁴ But He needed to go through Samaria.

⁵ So He came to a city of Samaria which is called Sychar, near the plot of ground that Jacob gave to his son Joseph. ⁶Now Jacob's well was there. Jesus therefore, being wearied from His journey, sat thus by the well. It was about the sixth hour.

⁷ A woman of Samaria came to draw water. Jesus said to her, "Give Me a drink." ⁸ For His disciples had gone away into the city to buy food.

⁹ Then the woman of Samaria said to Him, "How is it that You, being a Jew, ask a drink from me, a Samaritan woman?" For Jews have no dealings with Samaritans.

¹⁰ Jesus answered and said to her, "If you knew the gift of God, and who it is who says to you, 'Give Me a drink,' you would have asked Him, and He would have given you living water."

¹¹ The woman said to Him, "Sir, You have nothing to draw with, and the well is deep. Where then do You get that living water? ¹² Are You greater than our father Jacob, who gave us the well, and drank from it himself, as well as his sons and his livestock?"

¹³ Jesus answered and said to her, "Whoever drinks of this water will thirst again, ¹⁴ but whoever drinks of the water that I shall give him will never thirst. But the water that I shall give him will become in him a fountain of water springing up into everlasting life."

¹⁵ The woman said to Him, "Sir, give me this water, that I may not thirst, nor come here to draw."

¹⁶ Jesus said to her, "Go, call your husband, and come here."

¹⁷ The woman answered and said, "I have no husband."

Jesus said to her, "You have well said, 'I have no husband,' ¹⁸ for you have had five husbands, and the one whom you now have is not your husband; in that you spoke truly."

[19] The woman said to Him, "Sir, I perceive that You are a prophet. [20] Our fathers worshiped on this mountain, and you Jews say that in Jerusalem is the place where one ought to worship."

[21] Jesus said to her, "Woman, believe Me, the hour is coming when you will neither on this mountain, nor in Jerusalem, worship the Father. [22] You worship what you do not know; we know what we worship, for salvation is of the Jews. [23] But the hour is coming, and now is, when the true worshipers will worship the Father in spirit and truth; for the Father is seeking such to worship Him. [24] God is Spirit, and those who worship Him must worship in spirit and truth."

[25] The woman said to Him, "I know that Messiah is coming" (who is called Christ). "When He comes, He will tell us all things."

[26] Jesus said to her, "I who speak to you am He."

[27] And at this point His disciples came, and they marveled that He talked with a woman; yet no one said, "What do You seek?" or, "Why are You talking with her?"

[28] The woman then left her waterpot, went her way into the city, and said to the men, [29] "Come, see a Man who told me all things that I ever did. Could this be the Christ?"

How I Imagine the Rest of the Story: The Samaritan Woman Comes Home

You still here, Jim?

What do you mean? I live here.

No! You used to live here! You need to pack your stuff and go!

You're period on or something?

Sorry men always think something is wrong with a woman!

Maybe I'm wrong because I went to get the water I need from the well while you slept like a weak, fragile, helpless baby!

Maybe I'm wrong because I cook, clean, and care for a lazy no count like you!

Maybe I'm wrong because I thought you loved me but all you love is these Samaritan hips!

Yea, I'm wrong for being with your sorry, silly, stupid stealing snake of a boy!

Get out!

Why woman, why?

I met somebody.

Who?

You wouldn't know him cause he got a job!

He talked to me like I was a lady, not some Samaritan trash!

He made me feel like I was somebody special.

He listened and looked into my soul.

He showed me a look like I never had before.

What's his name?

Why you worried 'bout his name?

What's his name?

You don't need to know his name! All you need to know is that you ain't half the man he is!

Woman, what's his name?

All right! His name is Jesus and meeting him let me know I ain't got time for broke jokes like you!

The Widow's Two Mites

Mark 12:41-44 New King James Version

[41] Now Jesus sat opposite the treasury and saw how the people put money into the treasury. And many who were rich put in much. [42] Then one poor widow came and threw in two mites, which make a quadrans. [43] So He called His disciples to Himself and said to them, "Assuredly, I say to you that this poor widow has put in more than all those who have given to the treasury; [44] for they all put in out of their abundance, but she out of her poverty put in all that she had, her whole livelihood."

How I Imagine the Rest of the Story: The Poor Widow Walks Home

The tears ran down her face like springs of a waterfall. She thought to herself I never felt more embarrassed but at the same time I never felt more loved. Yes, the men bragged about how much they gave. They made sure everybody knew they had big money. They made sure everybody saw them as they reached for their big wallets. And they made sure everybody saw me. I'm the poor little sad widow. They might as well have shined a spotlight on me. Everybody saw all I had to give was two mites. I wanted to give more but my kids needed new sandals. My youngest needed a coat. Then I had to buy groceries. I'm doing the best I can by myself. I have nobody. I don't have no family. Since Earl died nobody, really comes around. I feel so alone. I was losing hope until today. I met Jesus for the first time and I know I can make it. I know he cares. Most of all I know he loves me.

Dorcas Restored to Life

Acts 9:36-42 New King James Version

[36] At Joppa there was a certain disciple named Tabitha, which is translated Dorcas. This woman was full of good works and charitable deeds which she did. [37] But it happened in those days that she became sick and died. When they had washed her, they laid her in an upper room. [38] And since Lydda was near Joppa, and the disciples had heard that Peter was there, they sent two men to him, imploring him not to delay in coming to them. [39] Then Peter arose and went with them. When he had

come, they brought him to the upper room. And all the widows stood by him weeping, showing the tunics and garments which Dorcas had made while she was with them. *40* But Peter put them all out, and knelt down and prayed. And turning to the body he said, "Tabitha, arise." And she opened her eyes, and when she saw Peter she sat up. *41* Then he gave her his hand and lifted her up; and when he had called the saints and widows, he presented her alive. *42* And it became known throughout all Joppa, and many believed on the Lord.

How I Imagine the Rest of the Story: Dorcas Gives Her Testimony

"Dead sleep is the best sleep."

"Praise God for using Peter to bring me back to life."

"I learned three things while I was dead."

"Number one, a dead woman can't help nobody."

Y'all know all the stuff I been doing. Helping the widows, volunteering at the Joppa Medical Center, and cooking for the church summer feeding program. Plus taking care of the kids cause y'all know my husband got a camel company and had to take a load fifty miles one way.

"Number two, I need to learn to say no."

I never have time for me. I'm always doing something for somebody but never doing anything for me.

"And Number three, I'm gonna take a vacation because y'all ain't killing me again."

You must have play time.

It was love at first sight. I was mesmerized by her eyes. She was beautiful, cute, and adorable all rolled into one baby. My first baby, the first half of my "Wonder Twins", my Alyssa stole my heart the first moment I saw her.

Hello I'm your daddy!

She opened her eyes as if to say I'm so glad to finally see you daddy.

I love you baby.

She immediately blanketed me with a feeling of love that made my knees buckled due to the force of her love.

I was standing but it was a love TKO and the fight was over one second in the first round.

I must admit that I don't do enough play time. My daughter, Suga has been working diligently to try to change that. She has taught me the value of play and she does her best to include me in it. Even though, I may be the most boring man in America my daughters still want to play with me. Suga is just a little more persistent. I am always fascinated with her creativity and her ability to make little crafts. She does so many things just for fun. She even cooks and bakes not because she has to but because she enjoys doing it. Often, I spend so much time doing things because I have to do them Suga reminds me that I need to do a few things just because I enjoy doing them and for no other reason.

Suga is so talented with her hands. She likes crafts, she wants to play soccer, and learn how to sew. Stacey and I cannot keep up with her always ready to do something fun pace. I thank God every day for giving me her to remind me life is not just about work, but life should also be fun.

What would Jesus Do? I remember the kids wearing the bracelets. This is an excellent question to ask when you are about to do something.

For instance, if you are invited to a party, ask yourself what Jesus would do. If you ask that question and you know that Jesus would not go, then you do not go. Would Jesus be in the club grinding with someone? You know he would not, so why would you try to do it?

The people that you attract will be attracted to you by what you do more than by what you say. Have you ever heard a young lady say that they always attract the wrong men? They say that they want a good man but pay attention to what they do and how they carry themselves. I know that there are always exceptions to the rule but generally their actions are attracting the wrong people.

I know that I have already talked about relationships, but I know that a lot of times you do recreation with others. Therefore, again the issue of choosing the right people to be around is important. You want to be with people who are striving to do something with their life.

Since you have a choice, please choose wisely. Regardless of the nature of the relationship, notice what a person does.

John 2:1-11 New King James Version (NKJV)

On the third day there was a wedding in Cana of Galilee, and the mother of Jesus was there.²Now both Jesus and His disciples were invited to the wedding.³And when they ran out of wine, the mother of Jesus said to Him, "They have no wine."

⁴Jesus said to her, "Woman, what does your concern have to do with Me? My hour has not yet come."

⁵His mother said to the servants, "Whatever He says to you, do it."

⁶Now there were set there six waterpots of stone, according to the manner of purification of the Jews, containing twenty or thirty gallons apiece.⁷Jesus said to them, "Fill the waterpots with water." And they filled them up to the brim.⁸And He said to them,"Draw some out now, and take it to the master of the feast." And they took it.⁹When the master of the feast had tasted the water that was made wine, and did not know where it came from (but the servants who had drawn the water knew), the master of the feast called the bridegroom.¹⁰And he said to him, "Every man at the beginning sets out the good wine, and when the guests have well drunk, then the inferior. You have kept the good wine until now!"

¹¹This beginning of signs Jesus did in Cana of Galilee, and manifested His glory; and His disciples believed in Him.

Top Ten Best Things about Being a "Girl Dad"

10) Your daughters give you hugs.

9) Your daughters give you love.

8) You get to love your daughters.

7) You get to watch your daughters grow up.

6) You get to play with your daughters.

5) You get to take care of your daughters.

4) Your daughters give you kisses.

3) You get to protect your daughters.

2) Your daughters give you their heart.

1) Your daughters steal your heart.

You can create your activities to do with family. If you are a dad, it is nothing more fun than spending time with your kids. I am working on spending more time with family.

The thing that helped me most was the fact that I knew on Sundays and Wednesdays that I would see these individuals at worship and Bible study, which encouraged me to go. Yes, we made mistakes but looking back I believe that I would have made more mistakes if it were not for my Christian friends.

It is important you find something that will help you relax in addition to your time with God. For you it may be playing basketball or pool. Or you may want to simply just like to hang out with friends.

Whatever you choose plan time to do it. Have fun in the mist of all the pressures of staying on top of your academics. Let the world know that there is fun in being a Christian. When I was in college, some of the most relaxing time was spent just hanging out at someone's house or a restaurant.

So, remember to have fun. Do not be fooled by the world that you must do the wrong thing to be entertained. You can enjoy yourself a lot more doing the right thing and I know if you have a good conscience that you will sleep better when you do right.

Remember God wants you to have joy. *Proverbs 17:22 says this "a joyful heart is good medicine." You serve a Savior who has been here on earth. Jesus understands you. No matter what you are going through.*

--Our Father,

You are loving. You are great. You are awesome. May we include you in all we do. Help others to know us as your followers by the way we love each other. Give us your Spirit to love when we do not want to love. Teach us to show others how to love us. May Your spirit fill us with Your love. In the name of Your son, Jesus we pray. Amen

Summary

- You must include God.

- You must get rid of bad habits.

- You must have play time.

Discussion Questions

1)   Are any of your relationships hurting you spiritually?

2)   Is there any sin that is in your life that you are holding on to?

3)   Would God be pleased with your recreational activities?

Day 3

Love Yourself by Loving You

My Credit is Falling Down

My credit is falling down
Falling down, falling down
My credit is falling down
My fair rating
Build it up with credit cards
Credit cards, credit cards
Build it up with credit cards
My fair rating.
Credit cards I cannot pay
Cannot pay, cannot pay
Credit cards I cannot pay
My fair rating
Build it up with a new car loan
New car loan, new car loan
Build it up with a new car loan
My fair rating.
New car will depreciate
Depreciate, depreciate
New car will depreciate
My fair rating
Build it up with more income
More income, more income
Build it up with more income
My fair rating

You must take care of your business.

"You should be ashamed of yourself."

"You don't care nothing about your mama."

"You go to church and sit up there and don't do anything about your mama."

"God is gonna get you for the way you treat your mama."

"Your girls won't visit you when you get old."

"Just wait and see they won't visit you when you get old."

"You gonna reap what you sow."

"You don't care nothing about your mama."

"After all she did for you."

"You don't care nothing about your mama."

The family member said so much more to let me know I was a sorry son, but my mind latched on to one phrase and would not let go.

"You don't care nothing about your mama."

"You don't care nothing about your mama."

"You don't care nothing about your mama."

"You don't care nothing about your mama."

"You don't care nothing about your mama."

"You don't care nothing about your mama."

"You don't care nothing about your mama."

It must have played in my head a thousand times each minute the family member spoke.

"You don't care nothing about your mama."

"You don't care nothing about your mama."

"You don't care nothing about your mama."

"You don't care nothing about your mama."

Immediately after hearing this I thought about all the times I would scrap money together since I was 12 to give to my mom. The times I sacrificed my food money to help my mom. All the late-night calls, the sleepless nights, the late-night drives to make sure she was all right.

I wanted to do more and at the time I should have been in a better situation to do more. But I could not allow anyone to say that I do not care about her. I just could not allow that to be said.

Then for the first time it hit me that I could live to be old and my girls probably would not come and see me. I was thinking yeah, you are probably right. I always just imagined I would be dead by age 45. I figured I would die from all the stress in dealing with my mom and all the hours I was working.

This was the first time that I thought that I may live a long time and be alone. I feel my life is about helping but I never could do enough for my mom's situation and now I was in a bad place financially and was not giving my mom what she needed. I guess that would be some type of poetic justice.

Luke 14:28 New King James Version (NKJV)
[28] *For which of you, intending to build a tower, does not sit down first and count the cost, whether he has enough to finish it—*

Miriam, my "Flash", entered my life as an extraordinary intern. Speed and proficiency is synonymous with her name. As my intern she kept me on task, which is hard to do. I tend to be all over the place. She helped me organize. She helped me become more efficient. She helped my get my act together. She completed everything with a smile. After the internship was over, we continued to talk periodically even though I was still all over the place. We became friends because we both had a deep respect for each other. Then she was hired as a case manager a few years later. Of course, I was ecstatic. She came to the team highly recommended by me and anyone else who saw her work as an intern.

As a case manager she is beyond outstanding. She is so efficient. One of the things that I noticed that she was able to do that I had problems doing was being able to say no. It didn't take long before the teacher became the student. I learned from her that you got to be able to not let people steal your time. For instance, if a person showed up late, then they would need to reschedule. I learned from Miriam that we must help people understand that our time is valuable. When people ask if you got a minute, are you busy, and I see you about to leave but Miriam could say no with ease. Sometimes she would help me out and say no for me.

No. It is such a short word but has such an impact. I notice that toddlers don't seem to have a problem saying no. However, as we grew up into adulthood, using this word appears to be a problem for some of us. Yet, one of my friends has taught me the value of saying no. Miriam taught me no is a complete sentence. Saying no helps to establish boundaries. Saying no frees us from unrealistic demands. Saying no gives our voice power. You got to want something better.

Saying no will give you more freedom to work on you and your stuff. Most of the time when I fail to complete something that is important to me it's usually because I overextended myself with commitments. Saying no is a part of a healthy lifestyle budget. This includes our time, our relationships, and it definitely has to include our finances.

Budget is not a curse word. Budgeting is saying no to unhealthy spending habits. You need a budget to manage your finances. Loving yourself includes not doing anything to harm yourself financially. You need money to live in this world. Do not destroy yourself financially by making bad decisions.

So how do you not be in debt while you are in school? Let me tell you what I plan to tell my children. I am not a financial advisor or financial planner. The best solution is to find a financial expert that can create a plan that meets your specific needs. However, this is the plan I would use for myself if I could do it over again.

In addition, if you do have a real emergency, instead of using a credit card you can use what you have in your emergency fund. Even if you must use all the money in your emergency fund, it is a lot better to start over saving at zero than be in the negatives because of debt. Once you graduate, I suggest you using Dave Ramsey's Plan in Total Money Makeover.

Also, take special care to protect your identity. Identity theft is real. Protect your social security number. Do not give it out to your friends. Be careful where you write it down. Be careful whom you give it to even if it is a business.

Secure all your credit cards and other personal information. Shred information such as bills or anything with your personal information on it before throwing it into the trash can. These are a few commonsense things that will help you to prevent identity theft. Do all you can to protect yourself.

You must take care of you.

Lightning struck my heart twice! Fifteen months later, again I was mesmerized by her eyes. She was beautiful, cute, and adorable all rolled into one baby. My Honey, my second half of my "Wonder Twin", my Alana stole my heart the first moment I saw her.

Hello, I'm your daddy!

She opened her eyes as if to say, "Really, daddy, you think I don't know who you are".

I love you baby.

She immediately blanketed me with a feeling of love that made my knees buckled due to the force of her love.

I was standing but it was a love TKO and the fight was over 1 second in the first round.

My baby girl, my Honey reminds me more than anybody else to take care of myself. "Daddy, you need to take a day off from work." "Daddy, you are working too many hours". "Daddy when are you coming home"? She calls me, she sends me messages, and she tells my wife that I need a break. She does the best job of anybody that I know of making sure she is taken care of.

Honey is not going to overwork herself. She will tell you when she is tired. She will ask for help. She will tell you that she is not a helper. Honey values her me time. Honey is willing to say what others may be thinking but afraid to say it. Honey has taught me that I need rest. She tells me, "Daddy you are working too much."

It is great to have a daughter like Honey who reminds you that you need to take care of yourself. Self-care is so important. We have to listen to our bodies and give it the proper rest, exercise, and nutrients it needs to function. We have to care about ourselves before anyone else will. Moreover, if you do not care about someone why would you take care of him/her?

Every woman has that one dress that makes her feel beautiful and this was hers. Not to mention she got more compliments on how good she looked when she wore this dress than any other outfit. When she put this dress on, she didn't walk, she glided. She began to slip the dress on beaming with confidence.

Then as she turned and looked in the mirror, she noticed that the dress was a little tighter than usual. It still sorts of fitted. But the dress was tighter for her because she always wore her clothes a little big. Did the dress shrink she thought? No, it' just been hanging in the closet.

She wondered what was going on. Then she realized that it might be her. She may have put on a few pounds but she never gained weight in high school so it must be something else.

Just to make sure and to prove to herself that maybe the dress shrunk or something else made the dress not fit, she decided to weigh herself. She stepped on the scale. Then, she looked down at the number. She was fifteen pounds heavier not lighter than she had been since leaving home for college.

Gaining weight can happen at any age. Let's think healthy and not weight. Let's start loving the skin that you are in. You are beautiful just the way you are. Your body is precious. Your body is a temple of the Holy Spirit (1 Corinthians 6:19). Your body is your responsibility. Take care of it because this is the only one that you get.

Since I am not a nutritionist or doctor, I am not going to advocate a certain eating plan. Consult with the professionals for the proper plan for you. I will say to use common sense in what you put in your body. However, there are a few things that I want you to consider with the acronym MOM (Moderation, Options, and Midnight).

Moderation is the key. You don't have to eat the whole pizza at one time. If you are not going to eat right, at least limit the amount of bad stuff that you are going to eat. Moderation may help you to prevent for packing on the pounds.

Options are another factor. When you have a choice, choose the healthier options. Maybe fruit for snacks instead of candy and chips. You may also be able to choose grilled chicken instead of fried chicken. I know that sometimes you don't get a choice but when you do, chose the one that is better for your health.

Midnight eating is something else to consider. You will be amazed at how many calories you may consume late at night if you are not careful. I am the type that I will eat whatever is easiest to get and I like to choose food where there is no preparation involved, which was often junk food. I later discovered that I would eat fruit instead of the junk if it were available. You may be the same way.

Your body needs rest. The body will only go but so long before it shuts down. Trust me I learned the hard way several times. Also do not forget to take vacations.

Top Ten Reasons You Know You Need a Vacation

10) You have two million seventy-six vacation hours that you could take off.

9) The last time you had a day off Regan was president.

8) You think working only forty hours is a vacation week.

7) You think when you work just one full time job, it's a vacation.

6) You work so many hours your timecard just says to be continued.

5) You think going to sleep during a root canal is a vacation.

4) You brag about never going on a vacation.

3) Your kids have to look at a picture of you to remember how you look.

2) You forget how to get home.

1) Your nickname at work is "Overtime".

Again, take vacations! Also, let's not forget to exercise and consult with your doctor for your personal exercise program. When you get to school, don't be a couch potato. You need some physical activity to stay into shape. Find ways to get exercise like walking. I also would take the stairs sometimes instead of the elevator. Even if you do not go to the gym, make some subtle adjustments in your lifestyle such as the ones that I mentioned. You can still be fit even if you don't have a lot of time.

1 Corinthians 6:19-20New King James Version (NKJV)
[19]Or do you not know that your body is the temple of the Holy Spirit who is in you, whom you have from God, and you are not your own? [20]For you were bought at a price; therefore glorify God in your body and in your spirit, which are God's.

We must remember the better you take care of yourself the better you are able to take care of others. Also, you will be better capable to do service for God. So, you must make sure taking care of you is a priority.

You must forgive yourself.

Her smile is infectious. As a counselor, I have seen her make sadness pack his bags and leave town. She radiates joy, sugar plums, cotton candy, and lollipops.

Alysha McConnell, my "Spider girl" captures people in a web of kindness. Alysha is one of the nicest people I know. She does her best to brighten everybody's day. She also taught me how to forgive. There was a person that we worked with that was not nice and very rude and condescending. However, what I saw with Alysha was her ability to love the person despite the person's actions.

It is so important to be able to forgive others of their transgressions. Equally or even more important is the fact that we need to be able to forgive ourselves. Consider forgiveness a present for yourself. Forgiveness sets us free of the bondage that shackles us.

Michael Jordan is perhaps the greatest basketball player of all time. Jordan had amazing talent. Jordan had amazing ability. Jordan had skills like no other. Jordan could hit shots that seemed impossible to make. But even Jordan did not make every shot. There were days that even his game was off.

The thing that amazes me most about Jordan was the fact that he could miss most of his shots throughout the game. Then somehow in the fourth quarter when the game was on the line, he starts making unbelievable shots and usually topped it off by hitting a last second shot.

Jordan had the ability to move past his mistakes and win the game.

We should learn from Jordan. The Bible says that we all have sinned and fallen short of the glory of God (Romans 3:23). Everybody makes mistakes. Nobody is perfect. Although, no Christian should use these phrases as an excuse to do something wrong, but when we do sin, we must remember that God provides a way for us to get back on track. He knows that we all have our flaws.

I have seen so many Christians become so paralyzed by a mistake that they leave God. When we do wrong, instead of leaving God let us embrace Him even more because His loving arms are still open to us. All we need to do is make things right with Him by asking him to forgive us.

We should learn from our mistakes. We all struggle with something. When we do the wrong thing, let us learn from what happened to prevent us from making the same mistake again. We should not linger in self-pity. Yes, we should feel bad about doing wrong. But we should not let guilt destroy us.

Sin has a way of humbling all of us. Sometimes Christian students are devastated because they did something that they never thought that they would do. They thought that they were so strong, but they succumbed to sin. Now they do not know how to deal with that.

So, as you have read the rules that were listed, just know you too are not so great that you too can't fall to sin. There are things that I did wrong because of my lack of knowledge. At the time I thought I was doing the right thing. And then there were times that I made bad decisions and I knew better.

I learned from all the experiences. There are times when you will make mistakes. When it happens, just own up to it and decide to change. Reflect so that you will know how to not to get yourself in that situation again. Reflect but don't dwell on the mistakes. You want to learn from mistakes so that you can move forward. You don't want to hold on to it because this prevents progress.

Do not let the thing you did wrong define you. Get back up and start to move forward again. Remember you are not the only one who has ever done wrong. The Bible says that all have sinned. Remember God is ready to forgive. All we must do is let Him.

Matthew 6:14-15New King James Version (NKJV)
14"For if you forgive men their trespasses, your heavenly Father will also forgive you.15But if you do not forgive men their trespasses, neither will your Father forgive your trespasses.

So how do you forgive? First, name the thing that you did wrong. Call yourself out and be specific. Ask God for help. Be sure to forgive others to be sure that God will forgive you. Make right the wrong if possible and go to the person that needs to forgive you if possible and ask for forgiveness the specific offense. Then be willing to give the person time and accept whatever response you are given. Finally, be willing to give yourself second, third, and one hundred chances and forgive yourself every time.

Dear Family,

Thank you for being a part of my life. Each of you are a blessing. I first want to apologize for my shortcomings. I have worked many hours and did not make enough money. I spent too much time helping others when more of my time could have been spent better my family. At times I failed to manage and monitor my own financials and failed to monitor my mom's affairs effectively. Then I allowed my body to fail me during critical times. I know you would have managed my life and my mom's life better if you were in my shoes. I made a lot of mistakes from age twelve until now trying to handle responsibilities. So, I ask that you forgive me, knowing that I did the best I could. Maybe I could have asked for your help more. Maybe I could have included you more. Maybe I could have been a better relative.

I hope that one day that God will give you the opportunity to say how bad I am, what a villain I am, or how bad God will eventually punish me for being inadequate. I would love to give you that chance but just not now. I just cannot give you that opportunity but just not today. There is just too much work that needs to be done and I must stay focused to do it. However, if God chooses to take my life before you are given a chance to confront me, please forgive me.

Know this, I have no animosity toward you, and I love and need you. Yet, right now I must focus on coming out of a bad situation. Also, if there is any way that you have wronged me, I forgive you. May God bless you always. Love, Abraham

You must be around good people.

I can remember when I was young, my mom used to tell me that she would not tell me anything wrong. She did all she could to instill in me good moral values. We did not have much money but she more than made up for the money that we did not have with her love!

There are so many good things my mom has given me over the years. But I believe the most important was giving me a strong sense of awareness that there is a God and that I should believe and obey him.

My mom used to quote this passage which was her motto for bringing me up. "Train up a child in the way he should go, even when he is old, he will not depart from it" (Proverbs 22:6). My mom did the best she could to train me to be prepared for this life and the next. All I must do is to take hold of the good that she gave me and continues to do so.

You will meet people who do not share the godly values that you may have gained at home. I beg of you to hold on to the good that you learned. Hold on to the good because your life depends on it. Hold on to the good because it will keep you out of trouble. Hold on to the good because it may be the thing that saves you from living a life of sin. Hold on to good people and surround yourself with them.

My mom gave me so much good. She also allowed good people to be in my life. I believe she knew that as a single parent that it was important for me to have a positive male figure in my life.

This person came in the form of a minister of a little congregation in my hometown. At the age of ten, I can remember wishing that my biological father was around, but circumstances did not allow that. I needed someone who would teach me how to be a man. God sent Brother Roland Cumbee.

My dad, Roland, taught me so much over the years. He taught me everything I know about the ministry and living life as a man. I have gotten so much good advice from him to take hold of. I feel that I can call him dad because he was there for me before I went to college. I can call him dad because he was there for me during college. I can call him dad because he has been there for me after college. And I can call him dad because I married his daughter.

Words cannot adequately express the impact Patrick Brooks has had on my life. He has been more than a friend. He is my brother. Pat has shown me love from the first day I met him. He is the one who taught me to drive. He is the one who allowed me to stay with him after graduating college. He is the one who has had my back every step of the way. No matter where he is he continues to be someone I can turn to and I am forever grateful that God saw fit to put him in my life.

Another great man God placed in my life is Brother Fred Sykes. Brother Sykes has been a mentor and father figure to me. I know there are certain things that I would not have gotten through if it were not for him. One of the things that Bro. Sykes has taught me to do is to take care of my business. He teaches through both example and suggestion.

He is very practical and frugal in his approach to finance. Some have even called him cheap. He was the first person to teach me about a spending diary and he had notebooks to show me that it could be done in real life. He talks about how you save money.

He still smiles when he talks about how much money he saved because he bought his outfit from Goodwill. He laughs when someone shares how much they spend in getting breakfast from a restaurant instead of cooking breakfast at home. He will wash out the aluminum pan when others toss it in the trash can after one use. He talks about how to live within your means. He has taught me so much about finances and handling your responsibilities.

Consequently, for seven years, I sat in a box called an office cubicle. For seven years on the other side of that cubicle was Terrence Gambrell. When you spend so much time in proximity with someone you either hate the person or they become your family. Terrence is my brother.

What do you do when your brother is on the other side of the cubicle? You learn about them. You worry about them. You want to help them solve their problems. You want the best for them. They show up when you need them. Anybody can talk about being a friend. Anybody can say they are your family. But your true friends are revealed when you are going through something. Terence was there when I was in need.

I must also mention the person that I can easily stay on the phone with for two hours. I must be incredibly careful because every time I get on the phone with my brother, Felix Weston. I can spend two hours on the phone talking about butterflies. Really, we can.

I believe, we think alike more than my other friends. However, he thinks at a quicker pace than I do. I think I may be more strategic than he is. He is the guy who usually gives me the most to think about. One of the things that I have learned from him is to always be willing to improve and get rid of bad habits. He constantly challenges me to get rid of some of my bad habits.

He reminds me that I need to sometimes get out of my comfort zone. He explains to me just because we did something one way for a long time does not mean that it is the best way. He tells me that education does not have to take place in the classroom.

I have received so many motivational speeches, videos, and documents. His honesty is refreshing in how he admits to still be working on certain aspects of his life. He is the first to tell you that he does not have all the answers. It is great when you have a person who you can just talk about anything and everything. Sometimes you need a release.

Most importantly, I must talk about the person that I have chosen to spend the rest of my life with, my wife, Stacey. We have been in each other's lives since middle school. She has shown me the meaning of true friendship and love. She is my diamond, my life partner, and the mother of my precious daughters, Alyssa, and Alana. I will always love them.

In conclusion, it is only appropriate to end by talking about a family like the "Incredibles." Brother Patrick Davis is a great man. He is someone who was there for me when my family and I were in need. He is someone that I respect so much for his actions. He and Sis. Lorraine have eight kids. They say behind every good man is a great woman.

This holds true with his wife Sister Lorraine Davis. Sister Lorraine Davis is an amazing woman. She is someone who can do it all. She is like "Elastic Woman". She is a great teacher, mentor, and friend. She has become a second mom. She has helped me when I was at my lowest. She has been someone I can talk to and she gives the best advice. She does not mind telling me I need to do something different. She has taught me how to love God and how to surround myself with good people. I thank God for putting her in my life.

As you can see, I need to make improvements. Fortunately, I have been blessed with great people around me. I just need to listen. Some men need a great woman to help them succeed. Apparently, I need a multitude of strong women to push and drag me to greatness. Also, I feel blessed to have only had a "heart attack" scare as the cardiac catheterization showed that I did not have a heart attack as the doctor thought.

Finally, I thank God for all the people, men, and women he has put in my life to be my guide especially during the rough times. Listen to the advice of the extraordinary women in this book. Mediate on what these superhero women say. More importantly, apply their words of wisdom to your life. Finally, remember that U Gotta Love Yourself!

--Our Father,

You are the wise one. May Your name be praised. Show us how to love ourselves despite our imperfections. Show us how to love the skin we are in. Help us to be kind to ourselves even though we make mistakes. Help us to forgive ourselves. Help us to love ourselves the way you love us. May You always be there for us and may we never let you go. In Jesus' most precious name, we ask. Amen

Summary

- You must take care of your business.

- You must take care of you.

- You must forgive you.

- You must be around good people.

Discussion Questions

1) Do you have a written budget?

2) What improvements can you make to take better care of your body?

3) Have you let guilt from past mistakes keep you from moving forward?

4) What have you learned from some of the mistakes that you have made?

5) Who are some of the people that have given you some good things to "take hold of"?

6) What are some good things that you have learned from people in your lives that you want to "take hold of"?

The Love Challenge

I challenge you to a love dare

A dare to commit to self-care

Please look in the mirror every day

And love every inch of you in every way

Remind yourself how blessed you are

You play the game of life like an All Star

Tell yourself I will take care of me

And that's the way it's supposed to be

Then say this phrase to everybody else

To help you I have to first help myself

Printed in Great Britain
by Amazon

28441781R00046